Bone Broth Power

Lose Weight, Improve Your Health, And Reverse Aging

Abraham Shilling

Respective authors own all copyrights not held by the publisher. The information herein is offered for informational purposes solely. The presentation of the information is without contract or any type of guarantee or assurance.

The trademarks that are used are without any consent, and the publication of the trademark is without permission or backing by the trademark owner. All trademarks and brands within this book are for clarification purposes only and are owned by the owners themselves, not affiliated with this document.

The Power That Is Bone Broth

Bone broth has the power to help us lose weight, improve health, reduce inflammation, and even reverse aging.

Loaded with nutrients, bone broth is one of the healthiest broths which one can consume. In this book you will learn all about bone broth and its powers. You will learn about its history, its nutritional content, its health benefits, how to use it to lose weight and suppress inflammation, and you should be implementing it in your life.

Many who have tried bone broth describe its effects as greatly improving the quality of their life, curing ailments of all sorts and as something that has no doubt had a life-changing impact on their overall health, happiness and well-being.

While the effects of bone broth, and the benefits it provides will vary in degree from person to person, it cannot be denied that its effects are nothing short of powerful, or dare I say ... magical!

If you haven't yet added bone broth to your diet, you just don't know what you are missing, not until you've tried it for yourself. This book will teach you everything you need to know in order to bring the magical force that is bone broth into your life.

Whatever issue may plague you, I would strongly urge you to not put off bone broth for another moment. It has helped many and in so many ways, that it's no wonder that so many out there are raving about it!

And you're in luck, because everything you've ever wanted to know about bone broth is right here, it's all in this book. All you need do is go through it.

I hope this magical elixir of power will forever change your life for the better as it has done for myself and so many others.

Wishing you lasting health, prosperity and happiness!

Introduction

I want to thank you and congratulate you for purchasing the book, *"Bone Broth Power - Lose Weight, Improve Your Health, And Reverse Aging."*

This book will give you a better understanding of what bone broth is, its benefits and how best to prepare it.

Healthy living requires that you maintain healthy eating habits because what and how you eat has a direct effect on your general health. Most of the diseases we suffer from today are because of poor eating habits. Most people prefer to eat processed food and sugar and this is why health problems like cancer, high blood pressure, and obesity are increasing every day. There is a need to be mindful of what you eat if you want to live a long healthy life. An example of a healthy and nutritious meal you should add to your regular diet is bone broth. For some of us bone broth may not be something new, while to others you may have heard about bone broth but you are not so sure what the fuss is all about. Whichever category you fall under, this book will provide you with more insight on what exactly bone broth is. You will also learn how bone broth can benefit you, how to prepare it, which bones to use as well as how to incorporate bone broth into your daily diet. Once you finish reading this book, you will have gained valuable knowledge about bone broth that can benefit you for the rest of your life.

Thanks again for purchasing this book, I hope you enjoy it!

Table of Contents

The History Of Bone Broth

Before we look at the history of bone broth, let us first learn what bone broth is. Bone broth is a meal that is in the form of a soup. It is made from simmering meat bones and meat scraps, usually beef bones, poultry bones and pork bones with a mixture of vegetables and spices. Bone broth usually requires a long simmering period, usually between 12 hours to 72 hours, and the heat used should be very low heat.

Bone broth has been used since the prehistoric era. It was initially eaten out of necessity, since back then there was no good hunting equipment, making it a very difficult task to catch or hunt animals. Therefore, every part of any animal that was killed was valued or used as food, including their bones and every shred of meat on them. It was unheard of to throw away any part of an animal because of the difficulty associated with hunting. The harder parts of the animal, for the most part being the bones, were kept on hot rocks in order to heat up, soften, and then break the bones so that they could later be eaten. A style of cooking with pots was later invented where the meat and bones of the animal would be put inside of a pot to cook for several hours.

The word 'broth' came from the German word 'bru' which means to prepare by boiling. The first place that bone broth was ever mentioned in writing was in an edition of the Dublin Courier in 1760. It was called a beef tea, and the paper went on to describe it as a hearty and healthy meal. Since then, this liquid meal has evolved and has been used as a health tonic, as an ingredient for food preparation, as well as even being served a warm breakfast. It later became a part of traditional Asian cuisine, for instance the Chinese ate it with vegetables to aid in digestion and cleanse the palate. In recent times, bone broth has become a major part of many healthy diets such as the ketogenic diet.

The Difference Between Stock And Broth

Many people, including myself, mistake stock for broth and vice-versa, because of the great similarities shared between the two. In fact, many people use these two terms interchangeably. Some of the similarities between stock and broth are that both of them are liquids obtained through boiling or simmering meat and bones together with spices and vegetables. Also, both broth and stock can be used as base for the preparation of gravies, soups, and sauces.

Some of the differences between the two are that stock requires the use of more bone than meat, but broth requires the use of more meat than bone. Also, stock cannot be served on its own as a meal, or at least it's not considered to be a meal itself; rather it is served as a base for making meals such as soups and sauces. Broth on the other hand can be served on its own, and is usually considered a meal. That said, broth can also be used as a base for the preparation of meals as an alternative to stock when stock is not available. A third difference between these two is the period required to prepare them. Stock requires a shorter period to prepare, which is between 4 to 6 hours. Broth on the other hand is easier to prepare but requires a longer simmering period to get the desired result. It generally takes between 12 hours to 72 hours to simmer bone broth, the magic that is bone broth occurs during this long simmering period. Finally, stock usually has a much thicker consistency than broth, while broth is usually more watery.

If you are at the moment in doubt of the importance of including bone broth in your everyday diet, the next chapter should make you into a believer, as it covers many of the healthy nutrients present in bone broth and explains its importance to your body, so do read on my dear friend, as all will soon be revealed.

healthy nutrients present in bone broth and explains its importance to your body, so do read on my dear friend, as all will soon be revealed.

The Nutritional Content Of Bone Broth

For you to understand the health benefits of consuming bone broth, you have to first of all understand what the vital nutrients contained within bone broth actually are, and how these nutrients are highly beneficial to the human body. Although there are over 20 nutrients and minerals present in bone broth I will discuss the most vital ones, and the role they play in revitalizing your body and health.

Glycine

Glycine is found in the meaty part of bone broth. Glycine is a non-essential amino acid. Some of the health benefits of glycine include:

1. Glycine is a type of glucogenic amino acid that helps to convert glucose into energy. This means that glycine is an essential ingredient used in the process of converting glucose in the bloodstream to energy used by your body's cells.

2. Glycine helps to create muscle tissue. It does this by boosting a compound called creatine in the body. Creatine is an absolutely essential ingredient in the body used for the building of muscle in the body. Yes, this is the same creatine you've maybe heard about, that bodybuilders take after their workouts.

3. Glycine is found in skin cells and its role is to firm up the skin cells. Thus, your skin remains firm even after being

subjected to Ultraviolet rays or after your body's cells undergo oxidation (the process of the aging of the skin).

4. Glycine aids in the digestion process because it helps in the secretion of bile acid, which is an essential acid for the digestion of fats.

5. Glycine assists in halting the function of the neurotransmitters that are responsible for depression, seizures, and hyperactivity disorders.

Proline

Proline is another vital nutrient present in bone broth. Proline is also a non-essential acid and is found in meat scraps. Some of the beneficial and essential functions of proline in the body are:

1. Proline helps to reduce the risk of cardiovascular or heart diseases like stroke, heart attack, and hypertension. It does this by reducing the build-up of arterial deposits that can cause heart disease.

2. Proline is essential for the production of cartilage in the body.

3. For the body's cells to be created, proteins have to be broken down inside the body. Proline facilitates the breakdown of protein so that the body's cells can be produced.

4. Proline combines with another amino acid called lysine to produce two other types of amino acids called hydroxylysine and hydroxyproline. These newly formed amino acids join together to produce collagen. Therefore, proline is essential for the production of collagen. We'll discuss the uses of collagen in the next section.

Collagen

Collagen is found in skin cells, tendons, cartilage, and ligaments. The amount of collagen in your body gradually drops as you get older. Research has confirmed that once a person turns 25 years old the amount of collagen in the human body drops at an approximate fixed rate of 1.5% annually every year thereafter. That is why it is absolutely essential that you include collagen in your diet. Thankfully bone broth is high in collagen. Collagen is important in that:

1. Collagen assists with digestion. It helps to break down protein and fatty acids for easy digestion. It does this by producing hydrochloric acid that helps in the digestion of protein.

2. Collagen helps to repair the mucus lining inside your stomach.

3. Collagen which is found in skin cells helps to make your skin firm and increase the elasticity of your skin. It also helps to regenerate and revitalize your skin, thus collagen can be said to be vital for slowing down the aging process because of the presence of amino acids in it. The amino acids in collagen responsible for slowing down the aging process include alanine, proline, glycine, and hydroxyproline. These amino acids act as a natural moisturizer, reduce wrinkles, and make your skin glow.

4. Collagen is vital for weight loss. A tablespoon of collagen contains over 9 grams of protein, thus it helps to keep you full and reduce your food intake.

Gelatin

Gelatin is derived when collagen is subjected to a hydrolysis process or extended heating process. Gelatin contains about 18 essential amino acids and every tablespoon of gelatin you eat contains over 6 grams of protein making it highly essential for the body. Some of the benefits of gelatin in the body are:

1. Although Gelatin on its own is not a complete protein it helps your body to break down and fully utilize other proteins you eat.

2. Gelatin also aids in digestion. It does this by mixing with water in your digestive tract to enable food to easily pass through the digestive tract.

3. Gelatin combines with other essential amino acids to speed up the production of cartilage in your joints. In addition to the role it plays in the production of cartilage, gelatin also contains anti-inflammatory properties that help to reduce pain and friction on your joints.

4. Gelatin contains keratin, which is a type of protein that helps to maintain healthy nails, teeth, hair, and skin.

5. Gelatin helps to boost your metabolism level and thus helps in weight loss.

Magnesium

Magnesium is another important nutrient you get when you include bone broth in your regular diet. Some of its benefits to the body include:

1. Magnesium helps to increase the level of melatonin. Melatonin is a hormone that is responsible for inducing sleep. When this hormone is lower than the normal level, the result is that you may find it difficult to fall asleep. Secondly, magnesium helps to reduce the stress hormone, cortisol.

2. Serotonin is a hormone that helps to relax your nervous system and put you in a happy mood. This hormone depends on magnesium to function.

3. Magnesium promotes strong and healthy bones. It does this by facilitating the production of Insulin-like Growth Factor-1 (IGF-) that helps in the growth of healthy muscles. In addition to the growth of muscles, magnesium helps to loosen up your muscles to increase flexibility. Magnesium also helps to prevent the build-up of lactic acid which is responsible for tightness and pain in the muscles causing muscle cramps.

4. Magnesium helps in the development of healthy teeth. It does this by balancing the level of calcium and phosphorous in your saliva, which in turn nourishes your teeth and keeps them healthy.

5. Magnesium allows free bowel movement by cleansing out toxins from the stomach. Thus, it helps to prevent constipation..

6. Magnesium is very important for diabetic patients. It helps to increase the secretion of insulin and makes the body's cells sensitive to insulin.

Calcium

Calcium helps build healthy bones. Your body absorbs calcium and uses it together with magnesium and vitamin D to increase bone mass. In addition, calcium is beneficial since it facilitates weight loss. It does this by increasing your body's metabolism level in order to burn or use up stored up fats, and this leads to weight loss.

With all the amazing nutrients that bone broth is rich in, it is definitely beneficial. Let us look at some of the amazing benefits you get from consuming bone broth.

Health Benefits Of Bone Broth

There are many health benefits of adding bone broth to your diet. Some of these benefits include:

It helps to improve digestion

As mentioned earlier, bone broth contains gelatin. Gelatin is a protein that is obtained from boiling bones, skins, tendons and ligaments. It contains a molecule known as hydrophilic colloid. Hydrophilic colloid holds digestive juices and helps to improve the secretion of gastric acid which aids in the breaking down of food into digestible bits. It also aids in the proper functioning of your digestive system.

It helps to promote healthy bones and teeth

Bone broth helps to strengthen your bones and teeth. This is because bone broth contains magnesium and calcium in very high quantities and these play an important role in the formation and strengthening of healthy bones and teeth.

It helps to reduce inflammation of the joints

When there is little or no lubrication in your joints, it will result in friction whenever you move, and this leads to inflammation and pain in your joints. This is what causes arthritis. Bone broth can help to reduce the inflammation in your joints because bone broth contains chondroitin, glucosamine, and sulfates, which are extracted from simmering cartilage for a long time. These compounds provide lubrication between the joints, and thus reduce inflammation and pain.

It helps to fight inflammation

Inflammation occurs in your body because of toxins that get into your body. Toxins feed the bad bacteria which then multiply to destroy the good bacteria. The result is a disruption in your body's balance and this leads to inflammation of the body's cells and also causes oxidative stress. Bone broth helps your body to fight inflammation because it contains amino acids such as arginine and proline, which have anti-inflammatory properties. Arginine specifically helps to cure sepsis, which is also known as the inflammation of the whole body. In addition, the collagen from bone cartilage turns to gelatin when you simmer for a long time. Gelatin contains glycine which is an anti-inflammatory amino acid.

It helps in weight loss

Weight loss is achieved when your calorie intake is lower than the calories you burn. Bone broth helps you lose weight because it contains very few calories. A cup of bone broth contains just 50 to 70 calories. Despite it being very low in calories, it keeps you full, thus making you eat less, and less food means less calorie intake. You can even lose more weight by going on a bone broth fast where you simply consume nothing but bone broth. Bone broth is rich in all essential nutrients so you will not be lacking any nutrients whatsoever. Since bone broth is low in calories, by consuming nothing but bone broth you are likely to lose a substantial amount of weight. You can do a bone broth fast for 3 days or even more.

It has anti-aging properties

Some of the main factors that speed-up the aging process are stress and toxins; examples are toxins from smoking, alcohol, and processed food. The Aging process is characterized by weak, saggy, and wrinkled skin. Bone broth can help to slow down your aging process. This is because bone broth contains collagen and when eaten, the collagen helps to strengthen your skin cells and slow down the aging process. Also, bone broth contains an acid called hyaluronic acid (which is usually found on a baby's skin) and the function of this acid is to hydrate your skin and remove wrinkles. Therefore, instead of spending money on expensive skin care products that claim to contain collagen, you should instead consume bone broth which will supply your skin with all the collagen it needs to look dazzling!

It helps to promote healthy hair

Many people who have included bone broth in their diet have confirmed that they experienced noticeable growth in their hair. This is because the collagen and gelatin in bone broth helps to promote growth as well as increase the radiant nature of human hair. It does not only facilitate hair growth but gives hair a shiny and silky texture. Therefore, if you have hair loss problems you definitely should make bone broth a regular part of your diet.

It promotes good sleep

Bone broth contains a sizable amount of gelatin, and ingesting gelatin at night before you go to sleep helps to promote good sleep. This is because of the presence of the amino acid glycine, which is found in gelatin. The function of glycine is to monitor and promote the effectiveness of the certain neurotransmitters which help to induce quality sleep as well as improve memory while in a waking state.

It helps to detox your liver

The major function of your liver is to clean out toxins from the body as waste. The liver is over-tasked these days, because of the overload of toxins that get into your body daily. These toxins find their way into your body through the food you eat, the water you drink, the air your breathe and even from the chemicals that are present in various body care products you use. The resulting effect is that your liver is overburdened as it works harder to ensure that toxins are removed from the body. If allowed to continue that way, it can lead to some serious health complications. Glycine, which is present in bone broth helps the liver to get rid of the toxins in the body. Thus, bone broth removes a great deal of the burden placed on your liver.

It helps to reduce the effects of the flu

The flu is usually characterized by a cold and fever. Chicken bones that you would add to bone broth contain a nutrient called neutrophil that helps to reduce the effects of the flu.

Bone Broth Diet

This chapter will discuss how to properly prepare bone broth, how to do a bone broth fast, provide tips for losing weight fast during a bone broth fast, and also provide advice on how one should add bone broth to their regular diet.

About the broth recipe

Making bone broth is not an exact science, so feel free to make adjustments to this recipe where you see fit and use this recipe as a framework for creating your own amazing bone broth recipes. Most of the ingredients in this recipe are optional, and you can experiment with it by changing the ingredients around, but most importantly you must add bones and meat for it to be bone broth (bones and meat are the only ingredients that are not optional). That said if you do follow this recipe exactly you'll get some excellent tasting bone broth.

The recipe (good for 3 servings)

Ingredients

1 medium sized onion

2 bunches of celery

1 tablespoon of ACV (apple cider vinegar)

¼ teaspoon of salt

1 pinch of pepper

4 pieces of chicken feet

2 lbs. of bones and meat scraps (your choice of what kinds to use, though cow, chicken, and pig bones are recommended)

1 garlic clove

Some spices and herbs (Your choice of kind and quantity, but I would recommend less)

2 bouillon stock cubes

Peppercorns (Your choice of amount)

How to prepare:

Wash the bones and meat, then mix them up with the spices. Place the meat and bones on a roasting pan and place them inside the oven. Allow it to roast for 30 minutes at a temperature of 350 degrees. Then remove the bones and allow them to cool for around 30 minutes. The purpose of roasting it is to make the meat tasty.

Then add the bones and roasted meat into a big pot. You need a pot that can hold about 5 gallons of water. Add water (just enough to cover the bones), ACV, and the chopped vegetables. Keep the parsley and garlic aside for adding much much later.

Bring the contents of the pot to a boil and allow it to continue boiling on high heat for about 20 to 30 minutes, then lower the heat and allow the broth to simmer.

After simmering for 3 hours, open the pot and use a long spoon to scoop out the foamy top layer.

Continue to monitor the broth and add water whenever the water level looks low.

After 10 to 12 hours, add the garlic and parsley, stir, then remove from heat. You can simmer it for a longer time if you want to (up to 72 hours). Remember that the longer you simmer it, the more nutrients will be released.

After you remove it from the heat, allow it to cool, then strain the broth into plastic containers and store it in the fridge.

Congratulations! You now have real bone broth, the stuff of magic! This broth can last up to 5 days.

Bone Broth Fast

A Bone Broth Fast, as the name implies is a type of fast in which you take only bone broth for a determined number of days. Nutritionists and dietitians recommend the bone broth fast for anybody who wishes to lose weight fast. Some people have confirmed that they lost almost 10 pounds for each week they were on a bone broth fast. So, how exactly can bone broth help you with weight loss?

How a bone broth fast helps with weight loss

I have mentioned that bone broth helps with weight loss; let us see how and why a bone broth fast aids in weight loss.

1. It helps to boost your metabolism: Metabolism is the process in which your body starts to make use of calories stored up in the body. Some of the nutrients in the bone broth such as gelatin and calcium help to speed up metabolism. When there is an increase in your metabolism without a direct increase in how many calories you eat, it will result in rapid weight loss.

2. Bone broth helps to cleanse your cellular matrix and this results in short-term weight loss. What it does is to release the fluid retained within the cellular matrix, and when the fluid is released, fat stores are broken down to excrete toxins from the body.

3. Finally, bone broth is very low in carbohydrates; therefore, during the fast, you can easily enter into ketosis. What this means is that if your body doesn't derive enough glucose which is the digested form of carbohydrate, it will start to break down fats which are stored inside the body to produce energy for body cells. Continuous breakdown of fats will result in quick weight loss.

In order for you to be successful while on a bone broth fast and lose significant weight, you will need a few tips. Below are a few tips to help you have a successful bone broth fast.

Tips for a successful bone broth fast

Prepare, prepare, and prepare some more: Before you embark on your fast, you have to make some adequate preparations. You have to decide how many days you wish to fast for; remember that the more time you spend fasting, the better the result will be. You can start out with fasting for a few days and extend it to a longer time-frame as you get used to fasting. Also, you have to prepare the broth the day before your fast starts, as it would be difficult trying to prepare your bone broth after you start your fast due to the long time it takes to prepare it. Since bone broth can last for 5 days, you should prepare several servings that will last for the time period you've planned for your fast.

Stay hydrated: Although bone broth is liquid, you need to ensure that you drink enough water during your fast. This helps to keep you energized, hydrated, and flushes out toxins from the body.

Add mild exercise: Engaging in mild exercise like yoga and stretching during the fast can help burn fat faster in addition to strengthening your muscles and body.

Adding Bone Broth To Your Life

While fasting is great, I actually recommend adding bone broth to your diet in your regular life, as it would bring you a myriad of health benefits. Ideally it would be best to consume bone broth once a day as a meal, although every other day would also be beneficial. Many have taken to drinking bone broth as their breakfast as well as myself, and this is what I'd recommend you do. If you have one serving of bone broth every day for breakfast, you will feel healthier, feel younger, lose weight, and basically enjoy a better quality of life where each and every day screams fun and excitement at you.

I should also say that your body will definitely thank you for adding bone broth to your diet, and your body will even tell you regularly that it needs and wants more bone broth! Don't believe me? Then go ahead and try adding bone broth to your diet for a week and you'll see what I mean!

Conclusion

Thank you again for purchasing this book!

I hope this book has enlightened you and improved your life. Adding bone broth to one's diet is without a doubt life-changing, and perhaps one of the best decisions that one can make in their life, so I highly recommend that you do so.

The next step is to implement what you have learned.

Thank you and good luck!

www.ingramcontent.com/pod-product-compliance
Lightning Source LLC
Chambersburg PA
CBHW061327250726
48657CB00003B/1080